# NO MORE TEARS;

## QUALITY
## OF CARE,
## LOVE, AND
## COMPASSION
## FOR THE
## ELDERLY

by *Dorothy Magliulo*

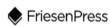

FriesenPress

One Printers Way
Altona, MB R0G 0B0
Canada

www.friesenpress.com

**Copyright © 2023 by Dorothy Magliulo C.N.A.& A.D.**
First Edition — 2023

Images used was from one resident that enjoyed doing craft while at the nursing home. I dedicated my book to my mom, she had cancer, she lived in her home while her daughters took care of her to the end of her life.

ISBN
978-1-03-917557-0 (Hardcover)
978-1-03-917556-3 (Paperback)
978-1-03-917558-7 (eBook)

1. MEDICAL, NURSING HOME CARE

Distributed to the trade by The Ingram Book Company

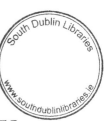

# TABLE OF CONTENTS

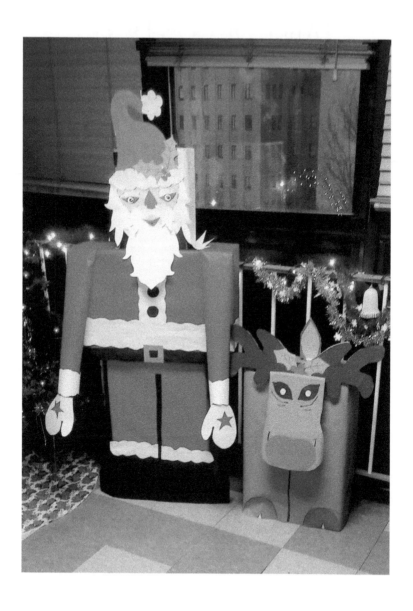

# Introduction

Despite some who go beyond their best in caring for the elderly, I have often found that nursing staff have forgotten the needs of elderly and to comfort, respect, and love them. When family members have no choice but to leave their loved ones in the hands of others in a nursing home, they hope their loved ones will be receiving the quality of care they require. The elderly almost never ask to be put into a nursing home—all they want is to live their remaining life in their own home. However, this is not always possible, so when they must live in a nursing home, it should be as much like their own home as possible. Unfortunately, in my viewing of nursing homes, most nursing homes have become more like institutions than homes.

This book is about my experiences in different nursing homes in New Jersey, first as a certified nurse aide and then as a Director of Recreation. In this book, I will provide information, my hopes, and dreams for nursing home care for an improvement for the elderly. You will also read on how activities provided to the elderlies are the best method for memory and quality of life.

# Working as a Certified Nurse Aide

In order for me to become a certified nurse aide (CNA), I first had to be certified within the state I live. I had to go to school in Jersey City for seven hours a day, for five days a week, while raising my four children.

For me, learning to become a CNA was so different than working in the real job force. In school, I was taught how to care for the elderly, how to be patient, and how to address them using the proper title of their name. I was taught how important it is to make sure the bedsheets are properly tucked in with a drawsheet, how to feed the elderly (e.g., a blind person needs more attention with food and direction on where the food is located), and how to take their temperature and vitals. I also learned how to transport the elderly from a bed to a wheelchair and a wheelchair to a bed using bedsheets.

While working in a nursing home, I was taught to call an elderly person "a resident" because they lived there. The clinical I handled at a nursing home in Newark seemed easy compared to my first job in Union City. I recall, in one clinical, I had to take care of three residents during my shift. One needed supervision in bathing while the other required complete care (meaning I had to do everything for that individual). The third elderly person had a medical condition in which he was paralyzed on one side and needed assisted bathing. The idea of helping the elderly has been something I've always looked forward too and am happy to attain to their needs.

## MY EXPERIENCES AS A CNA IN NEW JERSEY

When I started this position in 1994, I heard staff talk to the residents in a manner that made me question if I was in the right field. There was no respect for some elderly, who were belittled by certain staff. I saw no compassion, and some staff members never took the time to listen to them or even call them by their real name, only "mama," "sweetheart," and so on. If a resident wanted to stay in bed all day, the staff would tell them that they needed to get up, and nursing would instruct to us to do so. Bossing the elderly was something I had never expected I would hear or see. It was sad to know that people could be so mean to the elderly. I hope that I had made a difference in these elderly peoples' life.

My job as a CNA was such a challenge in the nursing home in Union City. I had eight residents to do within the seven-and-a-half-hour shift. I was never informed about a resident's condition, just given an assignment for the day.

My shift was from seven a.m. to three p.m. I gave morning care to the residents I was assign to. My job was to wake them up for breakfast, help clean their teeth and face, feed those who needed help, and pass out the trays of food together. When I finished with breakfast and picking up their trays, it was time to get them out of bed and placed in the dayroom (a room where they did an activity and ate lunch and dinner). Showering the residents was scheduled for once a week. The rest of the week, the residents were given a sponge bath, but some CNA staff would find time to shower their residents.

I was assigned a gentleman who had never let a CNA give him a shower or assist in washing. I went inside his room, introduced myself, and asked him if I could shower him or if he would prefer that I assist him in bathing. He allowed me to wash his body. During the process of washing him down, the wash cloth became so dirty that I needed more. He asked if I was trying to make him as white as me. I replied no, telling him I was only trying to make him look good and care about his appearance. He chuckled and said, "Thank you." Later, the staff asked how I got him to accept a wash from me. I said I simply went inside his room and asked him what he preferred, a shower or wash up?

After that, I was assigned another resident whom I knew nothing about. I knocked on his door and he let me in. I asked if he wanted a shower or help with bathing. As I gathered his clothes, he stood in front of his door and I was not able to get out. He pulled out his penis and started to masturbate. He told me I was beautiful and he needed to have me. I called for help, but all I could hear was the housekeeper man laughing outside the door. I was so scared, I took him by his arms and placed him on his bed, then ran to the nurse and told her what happen. She said she was sorry for not informing me about his condition. This nurse forgot to give him his shot, which was needed for his sexually behavior.

Then, I went into the room of another resident I hadn't helped before to do a.m. care. I took off his blanket and saw a giant tumor between his legs. I was startle and went to inform the nurse in charge. The charge nurse told me whenever I am assigned my residents, I need to go to their chart and read about their conditions. I believe the nurse on the floor should have informed me of the conditions of my assigned residents, as spending time reviewing the residents' charts would have taken valuable time away from each resident and the quality of their care would be minimized.

I was told by a resident that was given a shower, a CNA showered him from his head down, I noticed that this caused the residents' eyes to become bloodshot. (I went to that staff member about what she was taught during her CNA training.) Following that, when I asked a resident why was he screaming in the shower, his response was that the water was too cold. I informed the nurse on that unit, and she said that you cannot always believe each resident. The quality of care for this particular resident was lacking. When I reported this to the charge nurse, she replied, "You just started here;

you will get used of it." One aide had said to me, "We are swamped, with too many residents in a seven-and-a-half-hour shift." The facility felt that one CNA for eight residents was what the job description called for; it was part of the regulation from the state, I was told. At that time, in 1994, the pay rate for a CNA was only $6.50 an hour.

I left that facility for a job as a CNA at another nursing home in New Jersey, which was another experience altogether.

The first time I heard a resident crying, I went to see what was wrong. I knocked on the door and went in. I was shocked at what I saw. The CNA was slapping a female resident on the butt while she was bathing her. I asked the CNA what the hell was she doing, and she said she was trying to get the elderly woman to hold on to the sink so she could finish washing her down. I immediately went to the Director of Nursing (DON) and told her what I had just witnessed. The CNA was disciplined and that resident was no longer assigned to her.

When the nursing staff found out that I went to the Director of Nursing on behalf of the resident, I was called "the rat." This nurse's aide said to me, "You are the new person in the facility and what you see or do will not make a difference."

The following week, I was assigned residents that were too heavy to handle by myself. I had asked another CNA to assist me, but unfortunately, I was stuck with doing the care by myself. Another unfortunate situation happened while I was washing a resident from head to toe, as this resident was total assist. A nurse's aide came into the room and asked, "Why are you washing that resident from head to toe? The residents are schedule to take showers once a week." I was upset by that staff member's response and said, "Do you not wash your body every day?"

There was a lady brought to this facility who only spoke Spanish. She kept saying she wanted to go home and see her family in New York. When it was reported to the nurse on that floor, the nurse stated that she had dementia and was not going anywhere. Well, that resident escaped from the front door while there was a shift change and the staff had to go into groups to find her. Soon, the police were involved and the family became aware. Days later, the facility received a call stating that the lady made her way to New York with a fractured arm. The family decided to keep her close to home.

Another incident that occurred, I heard a female resident ask a CNA if she could put her to bed, but the CNA replied, "I am going on my break." I went to the resident and asked if she would like me to put her to bed. Although she was only ninety-six pounds, during the process, I heard a crack in my back, but I never reported it. The next day, I could barely walk, so I went to the DON and told her about what had happened to me. She told me that I could leave and go to the hospital. However, at the time, I was still waiting for medical insurance, so I told her I had no insurance. She said, "When this company pays you, you can pay your bill." This particular Director of Nursing treated her staff with no respect.

Unfortunately, I have learned that nursing staff never stand together to put an end to this kind of management behavior. They were too afraid to speak up for fear of losing their job.

During my time at this facility, I was assigned to the men on the fourth floor when the orderly who was usually assigned to them was off. I proceeded to wash each of these men and, while doing so, saw that their private parts were cake up with scum. One man had a lot of dandruff on his head, so I gave him a shower and cleaned his head so good that most of the dandruff was removed. After that, the team leader complimented me on such a job well done. I told her that I care for the elderly and love my job.

The following day, the fourth floor's orderly was very upset with me because the men there wanted me to care for them instead of him. The orderly went to the DON and told her I wanted his job. I got called to the office, where I had to explain myself. The DON preferred to believe him instead of me because he had worked there longer than me. The nurse on the fourth floor had to defend me; otherwise, I would have lost my job.

There was an older man who was put in a facility who never wanted to live in a nursing home. He had told his kids that he had a bad experience with his dad in a nursing home in New York. However, sadly, this man's family had no choice but to put him into a nursing home, as he was diagnosed with first stage Alzheimer's. While in the nursing home, he became combative and refused to take his medications. A nursing staff member called the family member in charge and informed him that his dad was combative and they needed his help. That son told the nursing staff that they could do whatever it took to settle him, so they gave him medication to sedate him. When his other children visited, they noticed he was so sleepy and was now in a wheelchair. A month later, this man died from neglect and unhappiness.

A woman was brought to the nursing home because her husband and children were not able to care for her at home. She was paralyzed from her neck down and was not able to communicate through speech. Instead, she used communication boards as well as the blinking of her eyes to indicate what she had to say. One day, a nurse came into her room and tried to give her medication. Using facial expressions and by moving her head, the resident tried to inform the nurse that she did not take insulin. Her husband came to visit and noticed that she was sad. She revealed what had happened that morning. Her husband reported the incident to Director of Nursing, and the DON followed through with an investigation.

Another gentleman was also accidentally given the wrong medication from the nurse. She had informed the DON and was told to keep an eye on him. A couple of hours went by. While a housekeeper was doing his job, he noticed that this man was not responding. He went and told the nurse, and sure enough, they had to call 911. This man was treated at the hospital.

Another resident that lived at this facility had aphasia and was paralyzed on one side of her body. One day, she was crying in pain and the CNA reported it to the nurse. This nurse stated that she would be right there. When her daughter came in for a visit, she saw her mom crying and called 911. Later that night, the daughter found out her mom had a stroke.

There was a man there who was on a feeding tube and he sat in a geriatric chair in his room until it was time for bed. When his son came to visit, he noticed that his dad was full of urine and his feeding tube was draining milk onto his body and bed. According to him, no one was aware of this. The son had a meeting with the nursing staff and a social worker about the care his dad was receiving. He was so tired of how the staff did not seem to care about the welfare of his dad. He had told them that when he had his dad at home, he had done a better job than the nursing staff and he wasn't trained. Unfortunately, he had to go back to work. He was so unhappy and hoped to see an improvement with the way his father was treated.

I had also witnessed several incidents regarding the social workers in the facility. When an older woman asked the social worker for her personal needs allowance, the social worker spoke to her without respect. In response, the elderly woman took the social worker's scarf from around her neck and tried to choke her. At another time, a resident had a container of milk and threw it at the social worker when she forgot to listen to his **request**. After the male resident choked the social worker with his bare hands, she felt he was not entitled to have his personal needs allowance anymore, which he had been receiving monthly. The social worker stated that he was getting dementia. When approached with this matter, she responded that some of these residents did not belong there and some were living at the facility for free. Those with no family were treated the worst, as they stood alone. Despite this, I had witnessed another social worker go above and beyond for the residents. She was a real advocate for them, but unfortunately, she left because the management had treated her wrongly. She was quickly replaced.

Once, I heard a resident ask to go to the bathroom in another language. The staff responded by telling the resident to speak English. However, even if a resident spoke English, often the staff would ignore them. In defense, some aides would say that these residents always wanted to go to the bathroom, or they would just let them pee on their self. When this resident asked the CNA to take her to the bathroom and the staff member ignored her, she got upset and decided to get out of her chair but she fell to the floor. When the nurse and CNA lifted her up, they saw that she was not lying—she was full of feces. That same resident received a hip fractured from her fall, and the family were made aware. In fact, there were many falls with residents that were left in the bathroom unattended, in their room, or in the hallway, or if staff forgot to put up their siderail while they were in bed, did not take the resident to the bathroom often enough, or left equipment in the hallway.

Some residents needed to be feed, but due to staff shortages, they had to wait. The staff would serve the residents according to whom they knew while the others sat and waited. Some residents would be feed rather late. When a resident lost weight, the nurse would call for the dietitian to improve their regiment.

If a resident voiced their opinion on any issue, they were called "troublemakers" and the staff would document on their behavior. This documentation would allow doctors, state surveyors, and others to read the resident's chart. Nursing taught medication was a good solution for behavioral residents.

I would often get upset when I had to care for too many residents within my seven a.m. to three p.m. shift. To do a good job, I knew I had to give up my two fifteen-minute breaks. What kept me going in this field, I reminder myself that one of the elderly people that I was taking care of, could easily have been my loved one. When an aide called out for that day, I would be assigned two more residents. In understaffed homes, residents were more likely to smell, including their breath, wear other residents' clothes, fall, or injure themselves.

The nurses of that facility hardly took the time to listen to some of the staff with regards to the residents' needs or wants. Nevertheless, there were some staff members there who really did care for the residents. I witness some staff members buy residents clothing and items they needed. Despite management telling them not to use their own money on the residents.

Once or twice a year, the social worker would call in a company to buy clothing for the residents. This company would charge high prices for items. Due to conservatorship, some residents did not control their personal needs allowance; instead, the company would use it for their clothing as they saw fit. It was so sad to see that their money was spent according to what the social worker and facility decided, and because the prices for the items supplied were so high, some residents received minimal clothing. For example, one pair of socks would cost $4; a house dress was $18; and so on. If there was more than $2,000 in a resident account, the facility would lose the resident's Medicaid. The social workers had to spend the resident's money any way possible.

## REFLECTING ON THE ROLE OF CAREGIVERS AND FAMILY MEMBERS

As certified nurse aides and nurses, we need to realize that elderly residents are in pain and their comfort is in our hands. If you are not capable of doing this job, I advise you to move on to a job that makes you happy. Remember, someday, we too will get old and someone may treat us as we have treated these elderly people. God wants us to love one another— search your soul before you hurt another elderly person.

We as adult children must be able to take care of our parents as much as possible before sending them off to a nursing home. The majority of parents were able to care of their children or child— now it is your turn to care of them. As from my point of view, some children don't take the time to care for their love ones. Remember, the elderly never ask to be put into a nursing home or put in the hands of others to be neglected. Know that elderly people do not want to be alone. Just because they may be ill or do not recognize you, that does not mean you should stop visiting them. They need you to have a voice for them, making a stand in making sure that nursing staff are doing a great job through comfort, love, understanding, and compassion . Also making the facility a home like environment and be there as much as possible.

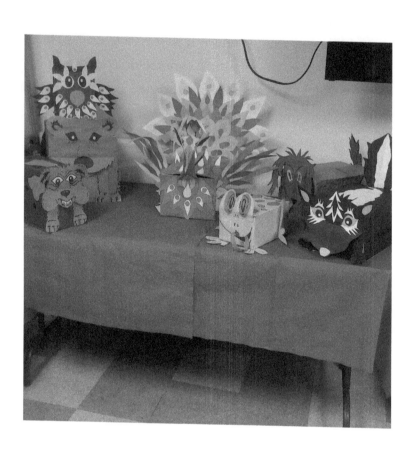

# Working as a Director of Recreation

Eventually, I went on to take the Modular Education Program for Activity Professionals 1 and 2 courses, along with some college courses in Jersey City. With all this knowledge, I became a director of Recreation at nursing homes in 2002 until 2018.

This new job for the elderly gave me much pleasure. In this position, I became closer to the residents and was able to give them a voice at the facility. I would listen to the requests they put together during the Resident Council Meetings, which were held once a month. Only for residents, these meeting were a place where the elderly could voice their concerns and inform each department about the issues that needed to be addressed. Their ideas were written down and distributed to each department for correction. I had to plan and put together activities according to their needs and interests. I spend a lot of time with the residents who needed a listening ear and reassurance. These meeting did help the residents; they had a voice when the management of each department listened to their concerns.

Some of the residents would come to my office and tell me what was happening at the facility. These residents wanted to chat and feel special. Some of the residents' issues, for example, were call bells not being answer on time, staff taking them out of bed too early, staff speaking to the resident disrespectfully, or the food not being tasty or cold. Sometimes breakfast was served late or some residents weren't getting their teeth brushed while others were being put to bed before dinner was served. Sometimes, their clothes were not theirs or they weren't asked which outfit they preferred to wear. Some residents had names outside their shirt while the clothes of others were being lost in laundry at the facility. Some were left sitting in their room unattended.

As the director of Recreation, I put some programs together to make a difference in the residents' lives. For example, the nursing staff and the social worker had put two residents together in the same room. The problem was that one resident was eating solid foods, while the other resident was on a feeding tube, as they were not able to eat anything through their mouth. Considering the resident who might be in danger if they ate solid food, I created a program which would avoid exposing them to solid foods. It was called the Personal Touch Program and was done during lunchtime. An activity aide would keep that resident occupied with an activity of their interest or capability in another room. This program was initiated for the purpose of all those residents who were NPO (nothing by mouth). Nursing staff did not realize what would happen if two people with different eating needs lived in the same room without special care.

The Recreation Department is there to maintain these kinds of achievements and be successful. The Director of Recreation and activity aides spend more time with the elderly than other staff members. We bring out their feeling through words and facial expressions. We listen, show love, and care enough to take time for them.

On a day-to-day basis, activity staff would ask other department staff to speak to the residents about the activity scheduled, even while nursing staff did their a.m. care. We were all here for one purpose: to give residents security, love, understanding, and comfort—and that's how it should always be. For us, teamwork went a long way.

## PROGRAMS FOR ELDERLY RESIDENTS

Delivering activities to residents depends on their cognitive level and capabilities. Certain activities are not for all the residents, so you must know what each residents' capabilities are before you engage them in an activity.

The staff must introduce an activity to each resident and explain how it is done. From my experience, if a staff member wanted to introduce a new game, it was best if they had it prepared and ready. If the staff had problems understanding the game, then we as a team would figure it out together.

You'd be surprise at how the residents would recall the activities, especially the ones they loved. We also had residents teach us some of the games they preferred, ones that we did not know. For example, they often enjoyed card games like Pitty Pat or Rummy, checkers, and chess. Once, we established how an activity was done, it became a memory for them.

The activity that seemed to be a hit with the residents with dementia and Alzheimer's at the facility was nursery, washing dishes, folding clothes, and sorting socks by color or size. The reason why these activities were such a hit was because most of the ladies were housewives and moms. If you sat with the ladies while they were doing these activities, they were able to chat about how many kids they have and the names of their kids. Sorting socks by color also helped them remember colors.

A popular activity for the Spanish residents at the facility was dominoes. It is a popular game that residents can play in a group setting. The residents could usually recall memories of when they played the game in their communities. In the summer months, the guys, and even the ladies, would gather around a table on their porch and play for hours. At the facility, we would usually have domino tournaments.

Some high-functioning residents would go on the computer to do research and play games such as solitaire and poker. Computers are a good resource to keep their mind intact. I also had residents who would look up movies from their native country. This is also another great reminiscing activity.

Working together with families is such a help for the elderly. In my department, I provided quality programs to residents that they'd enjoy, from bingo, checkers, dominoes, and card games to group discussions, birthday parties, and cooking lessons. We would have BBQs in the summer months, go to the store for them, organize church groups, and provide computers.

We held Activity Meetings with the residents monthly. They were the first ones to say they were pleased with the Recreation Department. Residents would also indicate the activities they wanted to do each month. Knowledge is the key in the ability to continue to improve a resident's quality of life. Getting the residents involved in as many activities as possible is a blessing. Through these meetings and through talking to the residents, we were able to learn the residents' interests so that we could format an activity to their liking and find out their diagnoses so that we could offer appropriate activities. Activity aides were there to focus on the residents' strengthens and needs. I myself had to review the residents' rights (F-Tags) of the Federal Regulatory Groups for Long Term Care Facilities.

I designed a schedule for activity aides from the time they entered the building to work (eight thirty a.m. to four thirty p.m.). It is important to note that along with the nursing staff, activity aides all should know the residents' name, call them by Mr. or Mrs., and always have their own identification visible to the residents. They should learn how to respectfully communicate with the residents and use communication boards when necessary. They also need to know who has falls diets, N.P.O(nothing by mouth). Activity aides should be well versed in all the Recreational programs as well as know what is each program.

Here is a list of programs for the Recreation Department, that was developed for the facility:

- *Exercise*: We offered certain morning exercises to the residents to help stimulate their minds and get their blood flowing.
- *Sunshine Club*: This program was for those residents who no longer able to do hands-on activities. The activity aide would work with their senses by providing sensory stimulation. The program provided comfort, triggered memories, and allowed residents to connect with others and maintain some form of movement with their limbs.
- *Mental Activity Games*: We used these games to keep the residents' minds intact for as long as possible.
- *Personal Touch*: We used this program for NPO (nothing by mouth) residents. In this case, the activity aide would provide the NPO resident with an activity during lunchtime to distract him or her from solid food.
- *Room Visit*: We used this program for those residents who preferred to stay in their room. Activity aides would visit them and offer an activity of their interest or preference. The aide would also encourage them to come out of their room from time to time.

- *Talking Book*: We used this program for residents who were blind or had severed impaired vision. A cassette player provided with different articles for that person to listen.

The purpose of each program was to help the resident:
- retain knowledge;
- feel that they are needed;
- look forward to something daily;
- feel comforted and recall memories;
- connect with others;
- avoid isolation;
- maintain movement; and,
- focus their attention, as in the case of the NPO resident, away from doing something harmful.

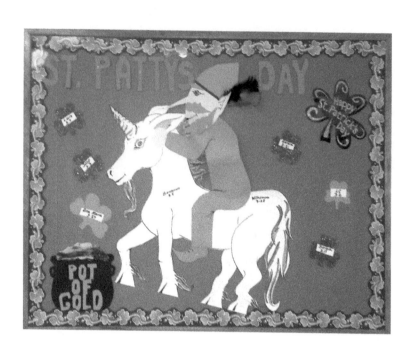

# What You Should Know
# and What You Can Do

Most nursing homes have an in-service nurse coordinator who sets up meetings to discuss different topics with staff in regards of resident rights, abuse, and so on. I have heard staff complain about the abuse happening at a facility. At a particular facility, the in-service coordinator, who had been doing the job for a long time, stated that she had heard this complaint. Her job would be to report it and go through the chain of command.

Firing a staff that harmed a resident through the union can be such a challenge for management. The union contract has three steps. You must verbally tell the staff, council, then write them up. During this process, there must be a union delegate present. If management only followed the union contract, maybe some of the bad apples would be gone and the residents would be safe. There are many nursing homes who have encountered lawsuits due to neglect and abuse. The union is for the staff and not for the residents. There is no one to fight for the residents, except for those family members who come often.

Social workers, who are the residents' advocate, often puts a blind eye to these matters. What I heard after we had a meeting with a resident and their family. The social worker would say the family feels guilty for leaving their loved one at the nursing home. Not realizing that the residents need us no matter what their issues, the social worker would say that some residents expected too much from us. She seemed to always have something negative to say about the residents, especially the ones who were homeless or on drugs. The social workers forgot what it is to have compassion and understanding for these residents. For example, when residents would go to her for help in finding an apartment, the social worker would tell them that they were capable of doing their own research. She had helped get rid of those residents who had a voice, were abusive, or were cursing. She stated that the nursing home was not a place for the homeless or drug users. I never seen that those residents were provided with other avenues to got to (example; counseling, support for their habits).

At a facility I worked at, there was an ombudsman that came during the Resident Council Meetings and sometimes on weekends. This was a plus for the residents, as any issues that were given to the ombudsman would be addressed to the administrator. I knew for a fact that management was not pleased when the ombudsman was in the building. The residents, however, would feel comfortable knowing that someone was listening to their needs and wants.

When it was time for state surveyors to come for their annually survey, the facility would work hard to look good. Each department head would come out of their office while the surveyors were there. At that time, the staff would treat the residents like residents and the food would taste better and hot. Nurses would be running around, making sure that the nurse aides were doing a good job. They would ensure that residents were not wearing other residents' clothing and were fed on time. Staff would greet the residents, be involved in the daily activity, and make sure incidents were avoided, that no equipment had been left in the halls, and that the facility smelled fresh and fragrant. We all knew when the state surveyors were in the building before, they even enter. There was a code they use on the intercom so everyone knew.

The state surveyors usually stayed for a good five days or longer, depending on what they found. They would investigate every department, focusing closely on the kitchen and nursing staff. Toward the end of their stay, the surveyors would inform the administrator of any deficiencies. A few departments could be without a deficiency. When a nursing home receives deficiencies, they are posted in each unit and the main lobby. Each person has a right to read the deficiency of any department.

I remain in touch with some of my residents through phone calls, visits, or postcards. I went to see one of the residents who was placed in a unit because he had tried to commit suicide with the call bell many years ago. While visiting this resident in Hudson County, I noticed his clothing and that he smelled of urine. I also saw a resident walk around with a crap stain down his jeans and another with a urine stain on his pants. There was a resident walking back and forth while another sang in the hall and one resident yelled at others. I saw residents sitting in the hallway, doing nothing. A male nurse was giving medication out as if he did not smell anything, nor even cared to see that these residents were not being cared for.

In the room of the resident I was visiting, I noticed his bed had no headboard. He did have the call bell on his bed, despite having tried to kill himself with one many years ago. His closet was locked and he had a TV only for show, as it did not work. When I reported this to the nurse on the floor, he said the TV was the maintenance staff's responsibility. This resident was alert enough to know that his quality of life was not even considered.

Residents are truly suffering from the hands of the nursing staff and the companies who run these facilities. The rooms in certain facilities are not fit for the elderly to live. Walls are cracked; paint is chipped. The walls weren't clean, cockroaches and fruit flies everywhere. The halls smell so bad that you want to vomit.

While visiting the residents in another nursing home in Jersey City, I asked an alert resident if they would like their picture taken for Halloween with me. However, a staff member yelled at me, saying I could not take their picture. I told this woman that these residents have rights and are alert enough to say if they want their picture taken. She pointed out the note on the wall stating no pictures allowed. I then said to her that she was violating their rights. The alert residents said she should leave us alone and mind her own business.

Many nursing homes around the country have problems with staff treating residents with no respect, no compassion, and no understanding and that do not take the time to listen to them. I truly believe that it all starts from the top, which is with management. If they valued the staff and their work, the staff may be more respectful, kind, understanding, and, most of all, loving to the residents. This would make such a difference in improving the residents' quality of life. I have witnessed nursing staff give medication and insulin shots to residents in the dining room in front of other residents. Where is the dignity for the elderly? The company only cares about getting their money on a monthly basis. They forget these are people who needed our help and reassurance.

## THE DIFFERENCE BETWEEN RESIDENTS AND PRISONERS

Prisoners have more privileges than a resident of a nursing home. Prisoners shower every day, while some residents shower once a week. Prisoners receive three square meals a day with taste, while residents receive three square meals without taste and with an unappealing look.

Dorothy Magliuloment>

Prisoners have entertainment, while residents' entertainment is monitored. Prisoners can stay in their cell, while residents must be out of bed. Prisoners do not pay rent; residents must pay rent with their social security money. Prisoners receive commissary in their account from family, while residents receive $35 to $50 a month for all the hard work from their jobs.

So, tell me, who has better life? The only thing that they both have in common—they live in an institution.

## WHAT YOU SHOULD LOOK FOR IN A NURSING HOME

For those who need help in finding a nursing home for your loved one in the state of New Jersey, here is some important information.

You must take a tour around the facility. If the place looks dirty, it means staff are not doing their jobs. Notice how the residents are dressed and cared for.

Speak to the Finance Department staff in regards to payment. If your loved one has money in the bank or owns a house, it belongs to the facility. A resident must be broke to get Medicaid to help with the monthly rent. So, before you put your loved one in a nursing home, make sure nothing is in her or his name for about six years.

Ask for the rights of the resident and review them with the social worker. Ask about your loved one's personal need allowance, who will be assigned to your loved one—the

30

CNA, the orderly, and the nurse on all three shifts. Find out who the supervisor is on all shifts, the director of Nursing, and the administrator.

If your loved one needs therapy in the three branches (physical, occupation, and speech therapy) as well as dietary help, look at the deficiency record of those departments for past years. Find out what activities the facility provides.

Make sure you inform the admission director, nursing staff, and the social worker who is responsible for your loved one in case something happens. Speak to the social worker on burial arrangements as well as who is going to wash and buy your loved one's clothes. Make sure they have an inventory sheet for all your loved one's belongings and get a copy of all the clothing that is logged in. Clothes can go missing, so this list is important to keep track of their belongings; otherwise, you will not get reimbursed.

The facility needs a phone number to be reached. Care Plan Meetings are on a schedule given by the MDS coordinator. The following staff involved in Care Plan Meetings: the nurse, social worker, CNA, dietitian, rehabilitation staff, and recreation staff. During the meeting, they will speak about your loved one's medical conditions, appointments, behaviors, doctors (who will see them monthly or when needed), food intake, and the activities they will be attending. The responsible person has a right to get copies of their loved one's diagnosis, medication, doctors information, and the notes from any Care Plan Meetings' held.

Even if the facility has a five-star rating, always be more involved with the facility you put your loved one in. When family members show up, often the staff pay more attention to that resident. Getting involved in your loved one's life helps them feel comfortable and not alone.

Here is some more information about resident's rights while living in a long-term care facility. The Nursing Home Reform Amendments of OBRA 1987 require that nursing facilities "promote and protect the rights of each resident." The resident's rights must be displayed in the nursing facility along with a contact number for the state's Long-Term Care Ombudsman (a third-party resident advocate). The F-Tags in the Federal Regulatory Groups for Long Term Care Facilities that may be of interest and know your loved one's rights:

- F550 Resident Rights/Exercise of Rights
- F551 Rights Exercised by Representative
- F552 Right to be Informed/Make Treatment Decisions
- F553 Right to Participate in Planning Care
- F554 Resident Self-Admin Meds-Clinically Appropriate
- F555 Right to Choose/Be Informed of Attending Physician
- F557 Respect, Dignity/Right to have Personal Property
- F558 Reasonable Accommodations of Needs/Preferences
- F559 Choose/Be Notified of Room/Roommate Change
- F560 Right to Refuse Certain Transfers

- Any F-Tags under 483.12 Freedom from Abuse, Neglect, and Exploitation
- F679 Activities Meet Interest/Needs of Each Resident
- F729Nurse Aide Registry Verification/ Retraining
- F730 Nurse Aide Perform Review – 12Hr/ Year In-service
- Any F-Tags under 483.60 Food and Nutrition Services

When the facility is not doing right by your loved one, file a complaint. The number is toll free (1-877-582-6995) or contact the ombudsman of New Jersey at Ombudsman@ Itco.nj.gov or write to: N.J. Long Term Care Ombudsman, PO Box 852, Trenton, NJ, 08625-0852.

With knowledge people can make a difference to the elderly. There are two pages of the residents' rights on Centers for Medicare & Medicaid Services website (www.CMS.gov). It has guidelines for those who often do not know about all their rights.

## SOME TIPS TO IMPROVING A RESIDENT'S QUALITY OF CARE

Whether you are someone looking for a nursing home for a loved one, it's important to know what activities are available to help improve a residents' quality of life. Specifically, this is a list of tasks for staff members to do with residents while they are sitting in the activity room and it should be posted on the bulletin board.

33

It is often hard to attend to all the residents, so this list can make a difference for them. Believe me, sometimes, it takes a lot of encouragement to get staff motivated. Nevertheless, the activity aide should encourage staff to become familiar with the items on the list. It's also a nice change of atmosphere and scenery to transport residents from one floor to another to participate in an activity.

In my experience, some staff will initiate an activity with the residents. For example, there was a gentleman who worked in the nursing home facility in Jersey City as a housekeeper. His job was to maintain the resident's room by mopping, buffing, and taking out the garbage. But on top of his job, he also spent time with the elderly, sitting with them to play cards or chess or watch old fashion movies while reminiscing. He would go to the store to buy them snacks or cigarettes, and he would give any clothing he grew out of to residents who needed it. He advocated for the residents.

Here is a list of dayroom tasks for nursing aides and staff:

- Take residents with wandering behaviors for a structured walk.
- Point out pictures in the hallway and see if they able to recognize what is in them.
- Look at the windows and describe the scenery.
- Give a hand massage to impaired and restless residents with scented lotions.
- Read an article in the newspaper, book, or the Bible and reminisce about similar events in their life.

- Play simple word game or puzzles.
- Toss a ball or balloon in a group setting.
- Dance with them.
- Give a back rub.
- Do craft with them.

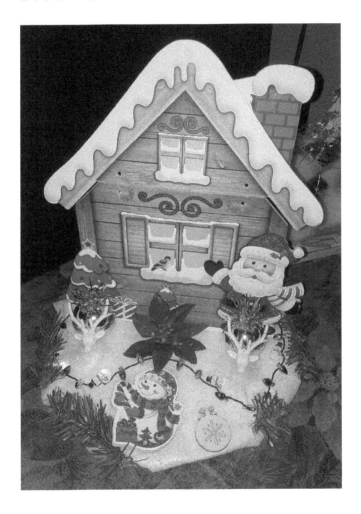

*An example of a craft using cardboard and construction paper*

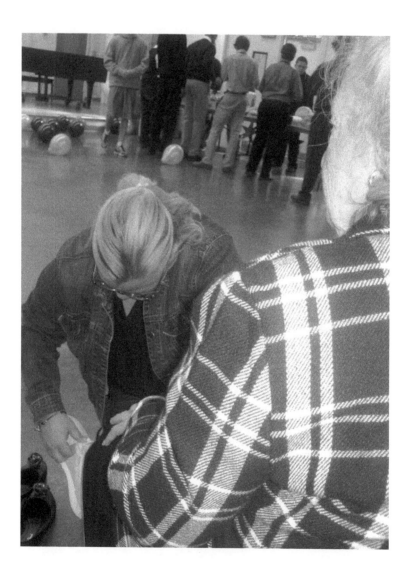

# Conclusion

As I sit here writing about the elderly, I find myself thinking, what happened to people today? Why is so hard for staff,
especially nursing staff, to care for the elderly? People just
care about their paycheck, not realizing that if it wasn't for
the elderly, they would not have a job. Nurses took courses
on caring for people in general—and the elderly are people.
I know that money is needed to pay bills, but so many do
not care enough to see the suffering an elderly person
goes through from the hands and words of others in their
nursing home.

When you take the time to speak to some of the elderly, you
will discover so much about them and what they have gone
through in life. It is like taking a history course. Most elderly
people never thought in their wildest dream that they would
be taken from their home to live in a nursing home, with
rules and others who treat them without respect and dignity.
With no color or homely decoration, with no comfort or
love, a nursing home is not a home—it is an institution.

If an elderly person has no family, their room at their nursing home so dreary. With the income the facility receives for rent, the elderly should live like they are in their home, with taste, color, and brightness.

When it comes to eating, they eat what is on the facility's menu for that day. Certain patients must be on a diet due to their medical condition. They often eat a big lunch and, for supper, a light meal. They eat lunch at a normal time—noon—but dinner is usually at four thirty p.m. The residents may or may not get a snack at night; it all depends on what the dietitian has written for everyone. How about those residents who are not able to feed themself? I saw a resident feeding another resident, due to the fact there was not enough staff or the nurses were too busy to come and help.

Residents are put to bed according to the staff's schedule. Some patients are put in their bed by the second shift (three p.m. to eleven p.m.) around four thirty p.m. If a resident wants to stay up late, they cannot because the next shift (eleven p.m. to seven a.m.) doesn't have enough staff available. Only ones that are allowed to stay up late are the well-behaved ones because the workers on the three p.m. to eleven p.m. shift do not want to deal with any incidents. The well-behaved are put in a recliner chair with "lap buddy" on them to keep them from wandering or getting hurt. If this is what an elderly must endure during their golden years, then God help us!

So much that goes on in a nursing home is pushed under the carpet or ignored. Shame on the companies that only see money and not people. Shame on the state who design regulations for the purpose of the residents but do not make sure they are being follow by staff. Shame on state for thinking that one person can take care of eight to nine residents on the day eight-hour shift, and one to twenty residents on the evening eight-hour shift. Shame on the families who dropped their loved one in the nursing home and only visit them during the holidays. Shame on the staff who prefer to stand alone and not fight together to make a difference for these residents, who have given us our paycheck. Shame on the companies who feel that the certified nurse aide does not deserve a good pay rate. Shame on the federal government that do not see that the minimum wage is not sufficient to earn a living. Shame on those people who think that treating the elderly in a cruel way is the right way.

God says to love one another. Treat others as you want to be treated. No one can predict when it will be their turn to be stuck in a nursing home. People should recognize that no matter what walk of life we come from, we all need each other. No one should judge others for any fault of the past. Being kind to others makes a difference, and following the state's resident's rights would improve the elderly's quality of care, which they deserve.

I learned a resident in a nursing home is the someone who lives there, but a patient in a nursing home is only there for rehabilitation before they return to the community.

## WHERE, WHY, WHAT, AND HOW: QUESTIONS TO ASK OUR POLICY MAKERS

Where is the quality of care for the elderly in the nursing home? Where does the nursing home care go from here?

Why does the company allow the abuse to go on in the nursing home? Why do the people who hire the nurses and CNAs never check that they are doing their job according to the well-being of the residents? Why do staff celebrate some holidays with residents before the actual holiday date?

What can management, nurses, and CNA do to make a difference for the elderly, to make them feel safe and bring them a home-like environment? What can we do to let them do something as simple as celebrate holidays on their actual dates?

How can management and nursing make a difference with change?

Each resident in a nursing home needs to feel like they are in their home and be treated with dignity and respect.

# About the Author

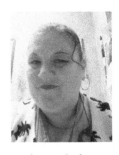I Dorothy Magliulo born and raised in Jersey City. I live with my husband Andre. A mother of five children. I have been on disability for three years, prior to my disability I was a Certified Nurses' Aide through the state of New Jersey, Activity Aide and than a Director of Activity. I went to school for two of my titles. One year of college at Hudson Community College in Jersey, took courses in person and online of Mepap 1&2 (stands for Modular Education Programs for Activity Professional). Taking theses courses helped me received my certification for Activity. Since I worked in the field of activity I love doing crafts, polishing nails, decorating, and most of all spending time with the elderly. This is my first book. I just want people to know what should we do for the elderly to improve the places of a nursing home. I want others to know, it should never matter where we come from on how one should be treated. The only award I received was the love and understanding of so many elderly. Until today I still kept in touch with the residents that were put into another nursing home by phone and cards send.

Ingram Content Group UK Ltd.
Milton Keynes UK
UKHW011302260723
425816UK00001B/62